The Ultimate Guide to Mastering Diabetes

Proven Strategies and Therapy for Effective Diagnosis and Management With Type 1 and 2 Diabetes Vitamins

Bhupen Thapa

Rollenkonflikt

Prioritäten setzen:

- Klare Prioritäten setzen und entscheiden, welche Rollen und Aufgaben am wichtigsten sind.

Zeitmanagement:

- Effektives Zeitmanagement, um die Anforderungen der verschiedenen Rollen besser zu koordinieren und zu erfüllen.

Delegation:

- Aufgaben delegieren und Unterstützung von anderen in Anspruch nehmen, um die Belastung zu reduzieren.

Grenzen setzen:

- Klare Grenzen zwischen den verschiedenen Rollen setzen und diese kommunizieren, um Überlastung zu vermeiden.

Selbstfürsorge:

- Auf die eigene Gesundheit und das Wohlbefinden achten, um stressbedingten Erkrankungen und Burnout vorzubeugen.

Kommunikation:

- Offene und ehrliche Kommunikation mit den beteiligten Personen, um Erwartungen und Anforderungen zu klären und mögliche Konflikte zu besprechen.

Den Konflikt als Chance sehen

Konflikte werden oft als negativ und störend wahrgenommen, können aber auch zahlreiche Chancen und positive Auswirkungen haben, wenn sie richtig gehandhabt werden.

Hier sind einige Möglichkeiten, wie Konflikte vorteilhaft sein können:

1. Verbesserte Kommunikation

- Offenlegung von Problemen: Konflikte bringen oft Probleme und Missverständnisse an die Oberfläche, die ansonsten unentdeckt bleiben würden. Dies bietet die Gelegenheit, diese Probleme zu identifizieren und zu lösen.

- Förderung offener Dialoge: Durch die Notwendigkeit, Konflikte zu klären, werden offene und ehrliche Gespräche gefördert. Dies kann die Kommunikationsfähigkeiten der beteiligten Personen verbessern und zu einem besseren Verständnis führen.

2. Stärkung von Beziehungen

- Tiefere Bindungen: Wenn Konflikte konstruktiv gelöst werden, können sie zu tieferen und stärkeren Beziehungen führen, da die beteiligten Personen lernen, sich gegenseitig besser zu verstehen und zu respektieren.

- Vertrauensaufbau: Das gemeinsame Lösen von Konflikten kann das Vertrauen zwischen den beteiligten Parteien stärken, da sie sehen, dass sie auch schwierige Situationen gemeinsam bewältigen können.

3. Persönliches Wachstum

- Selbstreflexion: Konflikte bieten die Möglichkeit zur Selbstreflexion. Sie zwingen uns, unsere eigenen Verhaltensweisen, Überzeugungen und Reaktionen zu überdenken und gegebenenfalls zu ändern.

- Entwicklung von Problemlösungsfähigkeiten: Der Umgang mit Konflikten kann unsere Fähigkeit zur Problemlösung verbessern, da wir lernen, kreative und effektive Lösungen zu finden.

4. Förderung von Innovation und Kreativität

- Neue Perspektiven: Konflikte bringen oft unterschiedliche Perspektiven und Ideen ans Licht, die zur Entwicklung innovativer Lösungen führen können.

- Kreative Lösungen: Die Notwendigkeit, Kompromisse zu finden und divergierende Ansichten zu integrieren, kann kreative Denkprozesse anregen und zu einzigartigen Lösungsansätzen führen.

5. Verbesserung der Teamdynamik

- Klarheit über Rollen und Erwartungen: Konflikte im Team können dazu führen, dass Rollen und Erwartungen klarer definiert und besser kommuniziert werden.

- Stärkere Zusammenarbeit: Durch die gemeinsame Bewältigung von Konflikten kann der Teamzusammenhalt gestärkt werden, was zu einer effizienteren und harmonischeren Zusammenarbeit führt.

6. Steigerung der Leistungsfähigkeit

- Motivation: Konflikte können als Katalysator für Veränderungen dienen, die zu einer verbesserten Arbeitsleistung und höheren Effizienz führen.

- Qualitätsverbesserung: Das Ansprechen und Lösen von Konflikten kann dazu beitragen, Prozesse und Abläufe zu verbessern, was zu einer höheren Qualität der Ergebnisse führt.

7. Förderung von Resilienz

- Stärkung der Belastbarkeit: Der Umgang mit Konflikten kann die Resilienz und Belastbarkeit der beteiligten Personen erhöhen, da sie lernen, mit Stress und Herausforderungen umzugehen.

- Erweiterung des Erfahrungsrepertoires: Jede konfliktbeladene Situation erweitert das Erfahrungsrepertoire und hilft, zukünftige Konflikte besser zu bewältigen.

Konflikte bieten zahlreiche Chancen für persönliches und berufliches Wachstum, verbesserte Kommunikation, stärkere Beziehungen und erhöhte Leistungsfähigkeit. Der Schlüssel liegt darin, Konflikte konstruktiv und lösungsorientiert anzugehen. Indem wir Konflikte als Gelegenheiten zur Verbesserung und Entwicklung sehen, können wir von den positiven Aspekten profitieren und langfristig gestärkt aus ihnen hervorgehen.

Nachwort

Konflikte sind ein unvermeidlicher Bestandteil des menschlichen Zusammenlebens. Sie treten in vielen Bereichen unseres Lebens auf – in der Familie, am Arbeitsplatz, in der Gemeinschaft und im globalen Kontext.

Obwohl Konflikte oft als störend und unangenehm empfunden werden, bieten sie auch eine einzigartige Gelegenheit für persönliches Wachstum, verbesserte Beziehungen und organisatorische Verbesserungen.

In diesem Buch haben wir die verschiedenen Facetten von Konflikten beleuchtet – von ihrer Definition und den unterschiedlichen Arten bis hin zu den Ursachen und Strategien zur Konfliktbewältigung. Wir haben erkannt, dass Konflikte, wenn sie konstruktiv gehandhabt werden, wertvolle Erkenntnisse und positive Veränderungen hervorbringen können.

Reflexion und Perspektive

Konflikte zwingen uns, unsere eigenen Werte, Überzeugungen und Verhaltensweisen zu hinterfragen. Sie fordern uns heraus, über den Tellerrand hinauszuschauen und die Perspektiven anderer zu verstehen. Diese Reflexion und Erweiterung des Horizonts sind wesentliche Schritte auf dem Weg zu persönlicher Reife und Weisheit.

Kommunikation als Schlüssel

Eine der wichtigsten Erkenntnisse dieses Buches ist die zentrale Rolle der Kommunikation bei der Konfliktbewältigung. Offenheit, Ehrlichkeit und Empathie sind unerlässlich, um Missverständnisse zu klären und Lösungen zu finden. Durch die Verbesserung unserer Kommunikationsfähigkeiten können wir nicht nur Konflikte effektiver lösen, sondern auch tiefere und authentischere Beziehungen aufbauen.

Chancen und Wachstum

Konflikte bieten die Chance, unsere Problemlösungsfähigkeiten und unsere Kreativität zu stärken. Sie fördern Innovation und Anpassungsfähigkeit, indem sie uns zwingen, neue Wege zu finden und kreative Lösungen zu entwickeln. In der beruflichen Umgebung können konstruktiv gelöste Konflikte zu einem stärkeren Teamgeist und einer höheren Leistungsfähigkeit führen.

Table of Content

CHAPTER 1

Understanding Diabetes

What is Diabetes?

Diabetes is a chronic condition that affects the way your body processes blood sugar, also known as glucose. There are two main types of diabetes: type 1 and type 2. Type 1 diabetes is an autoimmune disease where the body attacks and destroys insulin-producing cells in the pancreas. This results in a lack of insulin, the hormone responsible for regulating blood sugar levels. Type 2 diabetes, on the other hand, is characterized by insulin resistance, where the body's cells do not respond properly to insulin. This leads to high blood sugar levels and can eventually cause damage to organs and tissues in the body.

Having diabetes means that you must closely monitor your blood sugar levels and take steps to keep them within a healthy range. This typically involves a combination of medication, diet, exercise, and lifestyle modifications. By effectively managing your diabetes, you can reduce the risk of complications such as heart disease, stroke, kidney failure, and nerve damage.

One key aspect of managing diabetes is understanding the role of carbohydrates in your diet. Carbohydrates are the main source of energy for your body, but they can also cause blood sugar levels to spike if not consumed in moderation. It is important for individuals with diabetes to monitor their carbohydrate intake and choose healthy, complex carbohydrates such as whole grains, fruits, and vegetables over simple sugars and processed foods.

Regular physical activity is another essential component of effective diabetes management. Exercise helps to lower blood sugar levels, improve insulin sensitivity, and maintain a healthy weight. It is recommended that individuals with diabetes engage in a combination of aerobic exercise, strength training, and flexibility exercises on a regular basis to help control their blood sugar levels and reduce the risk of complications.

In conclusion, diabetes is a complex condition that requires careful monitoring and management. By understanding the basics of diabetes, including the different types, the role of carbohydrates in the diet, and the importance of regular exercise, individuals can take control of their health and reduce the risk of complications associated with diabetes. With the right strategies and support, mastering diabetes is possible for anyone looking to live a healthy and fulfilling life.

Types of Diabetes

Diabetes is a complex condition that affects millions of people worldwide. There are different types of diabetes, each with its own unique characteristics and treatment options. Understanding the different types of diabetes is crucial for effective diagnosis and management. In this chapter, we will explore the various types of diabetes and how they can be effectively managed.

Type 1 diabetes is an autoimmune condition in which the body's immune system attacks and destroys the insulin-producing cells in the pancreas. This results in a lack of insulin, the hormone that regulates blood sugar levels. People with type 1 diabetes require daily insulin injections to survive. Type 1 diabetes is typically diagnosed in childhood or adolescence, although it can occur at any age.

Type 2 diabetes is the most common form of diabetes and is characterized by insulin resistance, where the body's cells do not respond properly to insulin. This results in elevated blood sugar levels. Type 2 diabetes is often linked to lifestyle factors such as obesity, lack of physical activity, and poor diet. Treatment for type 2 diabetes may include oral medications, insulin therapy, and lifestyle changes such as diet and exercise.

Gestational diabetes occurs during pregnancy and is characterized by high blood sugar levels that develop during pregnancy. Gestational diabetes usually resolves after giving birth, but women who have had gestational diabetes are at an increased risk of developing type 2 diabetes later in life. Management of gestational diabetes may include blood sugar monitoring, diet and exercise, and insulin therapy if needed.

Other less common types of diabetes include MODY (Maturity-Onset Diabetes of the Young), which is a genetic form of diabetes that is often diagnosed in children or young adults. There is also LADA (Latent Autoimmune Diabetes in Adults), a form of diabetes that shares characteristics of both type 1 and type 2 diabetes. Understanding the different types of diabetes is essential for effective diagnosis and management. By working closely with healthcare providers and following a personalized treatment plan, individuals with diabetes can lead healthy and fulfilling lives.

Causes of Diabetes

Diabetes is a chronic condition that affects millions of people worldwide. Understanding the causes of diabetes is crucial for effectively managing the condition and improving overall health. There are several factors that can contribute to the development of diabetes, including genetics, lifestyle choices, and environmental factors.

One of the primary causes of diabetes is genetics. If you have a family history of diabetes, you may be at a higher risk of developing the condition yourself. Certain genes can make individuals more susceptible to diabetes, but genetics alone are not enough to cause diabetes. Lifestyle choices also play a significant role in the development of diabetes.

Poor diet and lack of physical activity are major risk factors for diabetes. Consuming high amounts of processed foods, sugary beverages, and unhealthy fats can lead to weight gain and insulin resistance, increasing the risk of developing type 2 diabetes. Additionally, a sedentary lifestyle can further exacerbate these risk factors, making it essential to maintain a healthy diet and engage in regular physical activity to prevent and manage diabetes.

Environmental factors can also contribute to the development of diabetes. Exposure to toxins, such as air pollution and certain chemicals, can increase the risk of developing diabetes.Additionally, stress and lack of sleep can impact blood sugar levels and insulin sensitivity, making it important to manage stress and prioritize healthy sleep habits to reduce the risk of diabetes.

In conclusion, understanding the causes of diabetes is key to effectively managing the condition and improving overall health. Genetics, lifestyle choices, and environmental factors all play a role in the development of diabetes, making it essential to make healthy choices and take proactive steps to prevent and manage the condition. By addressing these factors and working with healthcare professionals, individuals can take control of their diabetes and lead healthier, happier lives.

CHAPTER : 2

Vitamins for Type 1 and Type 2 Diabetes: Enhancing Health and Well-Being

Understanding Diabetes and the Role of Vitamins

Diabetes, both Type 1 and Type 2, affects the body's ability to regulate blood sugar levels, leading to various health complications. While Type 1 diabetes is an autoimmune condition requiring insulin therapy, Type 2 diabetes is often linked to lifestyle factors and insulin resistance. Alongside medication and lifestyle changes, a diet rich in essential vitamins and minerals can play a significant role in managing diabetes and improving overall health.

Vitamins for Type 1 Diabetes

Individuals with Type 1 diabetes need to manage their condition with insulin injections and careful monitoring of blood sugar levels. Ensuring an adequate intake of certain vitamins can support metabolic processes, boost immune function, and mitigate diabetes-related complications.

1. **Vitamin D**:

 - **Benefits**: Enhances insulin sensitivity, supports immune function, and promotes bone health. Vitamin D deficiency is common in individuals with diabetes and can exacerbate complications.

 - **Sources**: Sunlight exposure, fatty fish (like salmon and mackerel), fortified dairy products, and supplements. Regular blood tests can help monitor vitamin D levels and determine if supplementation is needed.

2. **Vitamin B12**:

   - **Benefits**: Essential for nerve health and red blood cell production. It helps prevent nephropathy, a common complication in diabetes.

   - **Sources**: Animal products such as meat, fish, dairy, and eggs. Vegetarians and those on metformin (a common diabetes medication) may require supplements due to potential deficiency.

3. **Vitamin C**:

   - **Benefits**: Powerful antioxidant that reduces oxidative stress and inflammation, which are heightened in diabetes.

   - **Sources**: Citrus fruits, strawberries, bell peppers, broccoli, and supplements.

4. **Vitamin E**:

   - **Benefits**: Protects cells from oxidative damage, supports immune function, and may improve insulin action.

   - **Sources**: Nuts, seeds, spinach, and vegetable oils.

5. **Magnesium**:

   - **Benefits**: Crucial for muscle and nerve function, blood sugar control, and blood pressure regulation. Magnesium deficiency can worsen insulin resistance.

   - **Sources**: Leafy green vegetables, nuts, seeds, whole grains, and supplements.

Vitamins for Type 2 Diabetes

Type 2 diabetes management focuses on improving insulin sensitivity and controlling blood sugar levels through diet, exercise, and medication. Certain vitamins can enhance metabolic health and provide additional support.

1. **Vitamin D**:

   - **Benefits**: Improves insulin sensitivity, supports bone health, and reduces inflammation. Deficiency in vitamin D is linked to increased risk of Type 2 diabetes.

   - **Sources**: Sunlight exposure, fatty fish, fortified dairy products, and supplements.

2. **Vitamin B1 (Thiamine)**:

   - **Benefits**: Supports carbohydrate metabolism and nerve function. Thiamine deficiency is common in diabetics and can lead to complications like neuropathy.

   - **Sources**: Whole grains, legumes, nuts, seeds, and supplements.

3. **Vitamin B7 (Biotin)**:

   - **Benefits**: Plays a role in glucose metabolism and can improve blood sugar control.

   - **Sources**: Eggs, almonds, sweet potatoes, spinach, and supplements.

4. **Vitamin C**:

   - **Benefits**: Reduces oxidative stress, supports immune health, and may improve endothelial function.

   - **Sources**: Citrus fruits, strawberries, bell peppers, broccoli, and supplements.

5. **Vitamin E**:

   - **Benefits**: Acts as an antioxidant, reducing oxidative stress and inflammation, and may improve insulin sensitivity.

   - **Sources**: Nuts, seeds, spinach, and vegetable oils.

6. **Chromium**:

  - **Benefits**: Enhances insulin action and helps regulate blood sugar levels. Chromium deficiency can impair glucose tolerance.

  - **Sources**: Broccoli, barley, oats, green beans, and supplements.

Incorporating More Healthy Vitamins

To ensure an adequate intake of these essential vitamins, consider the following tips:

1. **Eat a Rainbow of Fruits and Vegetables**: Different colors of fruits and vegetables provide a variety of vitamins and antioxidants. Aim to include a diverse range of produce in your meals to cover a broad spectrum of nutrients.

2. **Choose Whole Grains**: Whole grains like quinoa, brown rice, and whole wheat products are rich in B vitamins and fiber, which can help in managing blood sugar levels.

3. **Include Lean Proteins**: Foods like fish, poultry, beans, and legumes provide essential vitamins and minerals, and are important for overall nutrition.

4. **Opt for Healthy Fats**: Nuts, seeds, avocados, and olive oil are excellent sources of vitamin E and healthy fats, which are important for heart health and inflammation reduction.

5. **Consider Supplements**: If dietary intake is insufficient, consult with a healthcare provider about vitamin supplements tailored to your needs. Supplements can help fill nutritional gaps and support optimal health.

Conclusion

Managing diabetes effectively requires a holistic approach that includes a balanced diet rich in essential vitamins and minerals. By focusing on nutrient-dense foods and considering supplementation when necessary, individuals with Type 1 and Type 2 diabetes can support their overall health, improve their quality of life, and enhance their well-being. Always consult with a healthcare professional before making any significant changes to your diet or supplement regimen to ensure they are safe and appropriate for your individual health needs.

CHAPTER : 3

Diagnosis and Monitoring

Symptoms of Diabetes

Diabetes is a chronic condition that affects millions of people worldwide. Being aware of the symptoms of diabetes is crucial for effective diagnosis and management of the disease. In this sub-chapter, we will explore the common symptoms of diabetes that diabetes patients need to be aware of in order to take control of their health.

One of the most common symptoms of diabetes is frequent urination. This occurs when excess sugar builds up in the blood, causing the kidneys to work harder to filter it out. As a result, diabetes patients may find themselves needing to urinate more frequently, especially at night.

Another key symptom of diabetes is increased thirst. When blood sugar levels are high, the body tries to flush out the excess sugar through urination, leading to dehydration. This can leave diabetes patients feeling constantly thirsty and needing to drink more fluids throughout the day.

Unexplained weight loss can also be a symptom of diabetes. When the body is not able to properly use glucose for energy, it starts burning fat and muscle for fuel instead. This can lead to sudden and unexplained weight loss in diabetes patients, despite no changes in diet or exercise habits.

Fatigue and weakness are common symptoms of diabetes as well. When the body is not able to properly use glucose for energy, it can lead to feelings of tiredness and weakness. Diabetes patients may find themselves feeling exhausted even after getting enough rest, making it difficult to carry out daily activities.

In conclusion, being aware of the symptoms of diabetes is crucial for effective diagnosis and management of the disease. By recognizing the signs of diabetes early on, diabetes patients can take proactive steps to control their blood sugar levels and prevent complications. If you are experiencing any of these symptoms, it is important to consult with your healthcare provider for proper evaluation and treatment.

Diagnostic Tests for Diabetes

For individuals living with diabetes, understanding the importance of diagnostic tests is crucial in effectively managing the condition. Diagnostic tests for diabetes play a vital role in determining the presence of the disease, monitoring blood sugar levels, and assessing the overall health of the individual. By undergoing these tests regularly, patients can work with their healthcare team to develop a personalized treatment plan that meets their specific needs.

One of the most common diagnostic tests for diabetes is the fasting blood sugar test. This test involves measuring the level of glucose in the blood after an overnight fast. A fasting blood sugar level of 126 milligrams per deciliter (mg/dL) or higher on two separate occasions is indicative of diabetes. This test helps healthcare providers identify individuals who may have prediabetes or diabetes and need further evaluation and treatment.

Another important diagnostic test for diabetes is the oral glucose tolerance test (OGTT). This test involves measuring blood sugar levels before and two hours after consuming a sugary drink. An elevated blood sugar level two hours after the drink indicates impaired glucose tolerance or diabetes. The OGTT is often used to confirm a diagnosis of gestational diabetes in pregnant women and is also helpful in diagnosing type 2 diabetes in individuals at high risk for the disease.

Glycated hemoglobin (A1C) test is another valuable diagnostic tool for diabetes. This test measures the average blood sugar levels over the past two to three months by assessing the percentage of hemoglobin that is coated with sugar. An A1C level of 6.5% or higher indicates diabetes. The A1C test is particularly useful in monitoring long-term blood sugar control and guiding treatment decisions for individuals with diabetes.

In addition to these diagnostic tests, healthcare providers may also recommend other tests such as the random blood sugar test, the insulin level test, and the C-peptide test to further evaluate the individual's diabetes status and overall health. By working closely with their healthcare team and undergoing regular diagnostic tests, individuals with diabetes can take control of their condition and effectively manage their blood sugar levels to prevent complications and improve their quality of life.

Monitoring Blood Sugar Levels

Monitoring blood sugar levels is a crucial aspect of effectively managing diabetes. By keeping a close eye on your blood sugar levels, you can better understand how your body responds to different foods, medications, and activities. This information is essential for making informed decisions about your diabetes management plan and staying healthy.

There are several ways to monitor your blood sugar levels, including using a blood glucose meter, continuous glucose monitor (CGM), or even a smartphone app. It is important to work with your healthcare team to determine the best method for you based on your individual needs and lifestyle. Regular monitoring can help you identify patterns and trends in your blood sugar levels, allowing you to make adjustments to your diet, exercise routine, or medication as needed.

One of the key benefits of monitoring your blood sugar levels is that it can help you prevent complications associated with diabetes. By keeping your blood sugar levels within the target range recommended by your healthcare team, you can reduce your risk of developing long-term complications such as heart disease, kidney disease, and nerve damage. Monitoring your blood sugar levels regularly can also help you catch high or low blood sugar levels before they become a serious problem.

In addition to monitoring your blood sugar levels, it is important to keep track of other key health markers, such as blood pressure, cholesterol levels, and weight. Maintaining a healthy lifestyle through regular exercise, a balanced diet, and stress management techniques can also help improve your overall health and reduce your risk of complications related to diabetes. By taking a proactive approach to managing your diabetes, you can lead a full and healthy life while minimizing the impact of this chronic condition on your daily activities.

In conclusion, monitoring your blood sugar levels is an essential part of effectively managing diabetes. By keeping a close eye on your levels and working closely with your healthcare team, you can make informed decisions about your diabetes management plan and stay healthy. Remember that everyone's diabetes journey is unique, so it is important to find the monitoring tools and strategies that work best for you. With dedication and commitment, you can successfully navigate the challenges of diabetes and lead a fulfilling life.

CHAPTER : 4
Treatment Options

Medications for Diabetes

When it comes to managing diabetes, medications can play a crucial role in helping to control blood sugar levels and prevent complications. In this sub-chapter, we will discuss the various medications available for diabetes patients and how they can be used effectively as part of a comprehensive treatment plan.

One of the most common types of medications for diabetes is oral medications, which are taken in pill form. These medications work by either increasing insulin production in the body or helping the body use insulin more effectively. Some examples of oral medications include metformin, sulfonylureas, and thiazolidinediones. It is important to work closely with your healthcare provider to find the right combination of oral medications that work best for you.

For some diabetes patients, insulin therapy may be necessary to help control blood sugar levels. Insulin is a hormone that helps regulate blood sugar, and for people with diabetes who do not produce enough insulin on their own, insulin injections or an insulin pump may be necessary. There are different types of insulin available, including rapid-acting, short-acting, intermediate-acting, and long-acting insulin. Your healthcare provider will work with you to determine the right type and dosage of insulin for your needs.

In addition to oral medications and insulin therapy, there are also other medications that can be used to help manage diabetes and prevent complications. For example, medications to control blood pressure and cholesterol levels may be prescribed to reduce the risk of heart disease and stroke, which are common complications of diabetes. It is important to take all medications as prescribed and to follow up with your healthcare provider regularly to monitor your progress and make any necessary adjustments to your treatment plan.

In conclusion, medications play a vital role in the management of diabetes and can help patients achieve better control of their blood sugar levels and reduce the risk of complications. By working closely with your healthcare provider and following a comprehensive treatment plan that includes medications, diet, exercise, and regular monitoring, you can effectively manage your diabetes and improve your overall health and well-being. Remember, it is important to be proactive in managing your diabetes and to seek help from healthcare professionals whenever necessary.

Insulin Therapy

Insulin therapy is a crucial aspect of managing diabetes for many individuals. Whether you have type 1 diabetes or type 2 diabetes that requires insulin, understanding how insulin works and how to properly administer it is essential for effectively managing your blood sugar levels. In this section, we will explore the different types of insulin available, how to properly inject insulin, and tips for monitoring your blood sugar levels while on insulin therapy.

There are several types of insulin available for diabetes patients, including rapid-acting, short-acting, intermediate-acting, and long-acting insulin. Your healthcare provider will work with you to determine the best type of insulin for your individual needs based on factors such as your lifestyle, blood sugar levels, and overall health. It is important to follow your healthcare provider's instructions closely when it comes to dosing and timing of your insulin injections to ensure optimal blood sugar control.

Proper injection technique is essential for ensuring that you are receiving the full benefits of your insulin therapy. Before injecting insulin, make sure to wash your hands and the injection site with soap and water. Pinch the skin and inject the insulin at a 90-degree angle, being careful not to inject into muscle tissue. Rotate injection sites to prevent lipohypertrophy, a condition that can occur from injecting insulin in the same spot repeatedly.

Monitoring your blood sugar levels while on insulin therapy is also crucial for effectively managing your diabetes. Your healthcare provider may recommend checking your blood sugar levels multiple times a day, especially before and after meals and physical activity. Keeping a log of your blood sugar levels can help you and your healthcare provider make adjustments to your insulin dose as needed to keep your blood sugar levels within target range.

In conclusion, insulin therapy is a powerful tool for managing diabetes and maintaining optimal blood sugar control. By working closely with your healthcare provider to determine the best type of insulin for your individual needs, mastering proper injection technique, and monitoring your blood sugar levels regularly, you can effectively manage your diabetes and live a healthy, fulfilling life. Remember, diabetes management is a team effort, so don't hesitate to reach out to your healthcare provider for support and guidance along the way.

Lifestyle Changes for Managing Diabetes

If you have been diagnosed with diabetes, making lifestyle changes is crucial for effectively managing your condition. By implementing certain strategies, you can improve your overall health and well-being while keeping your blood sugar levels under control. In this subchapter, we will discuss some key lifestyle changes that can help you master diabetes and live a healthier life.

One of the most important lifestyle changes for managing diabetes is adopting a healthy diet. Eating a balanced diet that is rich in fruits, vegetables, whole grains, and lean proteins can help regulate your blood sugar levels and prevent spikes. Avoiding sugary and processed foods is also essential for maintaining stable blood sugar levels. Working with a registered dietitian can help you create a personalized meal plan that meets your nutritional needs while managing your diabetes effectively.

Regular physical activity is another crucial lifestyle change for managing diabetes. Exercise can help lower your blood sugar levels, improve insulin sensitivity, and reduce your risk of complications associated with diabetes. Aim for at least 30 minutes of moderate-intensity exercise most days of the week, such as walking, swimming, or cycling. Consult with your healthcare provider before starting any new exercise regimen to ensure it is safe for you.

Managing stress is also important for controlling diabetes. Stress can elevate your blood sugar levels and interfere with your ability to manage your condition effectively. Practice stress-reducing techniques such as deep breathing, meditation, yoga, or spending time in nature. Getting an adequate amount of sleep is also essential for maintaining stable blood sugar levels and overall health.

In addition to diet, exercise, stress management, and sleep, monitoring your blood sugar levels regularly is crucial for managing diabetes. Keeping track of your blood sugar levels can help you identify patterns, make necessary adjustments to your treatment plan, and prevent complications. Work closely with your healthcare team to develop a monitoring schedule that works for you. By making these lifestyle changes and working closely with your healthcare team, you can effectively manage your diabetes and improve your quality of life.

CHAPTER : 5

Benefits of Laughing Therapy for Diabetes

1. Stress Reduction:

- **Impact on Blood Sugar Levels**: Stress can lead to increased blood sugar levels due to the release of stress hormones like cortisol and adrenaline. Laughter therapy can reduce stress, which may help stabilize blood sugar levels.

- **Relaxation Response**: Laughter induces a relaxation response, lowering the heart rate and blood pressure, which can be beneficial for overall cardiovascular health.

2. Improved Mental Health:

- **Depression and Anxiety**: People with diabetes often experience higher rates of depression and anxiety. Laughter therapy can boost mood and reduce feelings of anxiety and depression by releasing endorphins, the body's natural feel-good chemicals.

- **Social Interaction**: Laughter therapy often involves group activities, promoting social interaction and reducing feelings of isolation, which can be particularly beneficial for mental well-being.

3. Enhanced Immune Function:

- **Immune Response**: Laughter has been shown to enhance immune function by increasing the production of antibodies and activating immune cells. A stronger immune system can help people with diabetes better manage infections and overall health.

4. Pain Management:

- **Natural Pain Relief**: Laughter triggers the release of endorphins, which can act as natural painkillers. This can be helpful for managing chronic pain conditions that are common in people with diabetes, such as neuropathy.

5. **Cardiovascular Health**:

  - **Blood Flow**: Laughter improves blood vessel function and increases blood flow, which can be beneficial for cardiovascular health. Cardiovascular complications are a significant concern for people with diabetes.

Scientific Evidence:

Several studies have explored the benefits of laughter therapy and its impact on health:

- **Stress Hormones**: Research has shown that laughter can reduce the levels of stress hormones, such as cortisol and adrenaline, which can indirectly help manage blood glucose levels.

- **Endorphins and Dopamine**: Laughter increases the release of endorphins and dopamine, improving mood and providing a sense of well-being.

- **Immune Function**: Studies have demonstrated that laughter can boost the immune system by increasing the number and activity of natural killer cells and other immune components.

- **Pain Tolerance**: Research indicates that laughter increases pain tolerance, likely due to the release of endorphins.

Example Book Titles on Laughing Therapy for Diabetes:

1. **"Laughter and Diabetes: Harnessing Humor for Better Health"**

2. **"The Healing Power of Laughter: A Guide for Diabetics"**

3. **"Laugh Away Diabetes: How Humor Can Improve Your Health"**

4. "Laughter Therapy for Diabetes: Scientific Insights and Practical Tips"

5. "Diabetes and Joy: Using Laughter to Manage Your Health"

These titles can provide a comprehensive view of how laughter therapy can be integrated into diabetes management.

CHAPTER : 6

Benefits of Breathing Exercises for Diabetes

1. **Stress Reduction**:

  - **Lower Stress Hormones**: Stress increases levels of cortisol and adrenaline, which can raise blood sugar levels. Breathing exercises help lower these stress hormones, promoting more stable blood glucose levels.

  - **Relaxation Response**: Engaging in deep breathing activates the parasympathetic nervous system, inducing a state of relaxation and reducing stress.

2. **Improved Blood Circulation**:

  - **Oxygen Supply**: Deep breathing increases oxygen supply to tissues, which can enhance blood circulation and improve the overall health of cells and tissues, including those affected by diabetes complications.

3. **Enhanced Insulin Sensitivity**:

  - **Regulation of Blood Sugar**: Regular practice of breathing exercises may improve insulin sensitivity, helping the body use glucose more effectively and lowering blood sugar levels.

4. **Better Mental Health**:

  - **Reduced Anxiety and Depression**: Breathing exercises can alleviate symptoms of anxiety and depression, which are common in individuals with diabetes, improving their mental health and quality of life.

How to Do Breathing Exercises

1. **Deep Breathing (Diaphragmatic Breathing)**:

   - Sit or lie down in a comfortable position.

   - Place one hand on your chest and the other on your abdomen.

   - Inhale deeply through your nose, allowing your abdomen to rise while keeping your chest relatively still.

   - Exhale slowly through your mouth, letting your abdomen fall.

   - Repeat for 5-10 minutes, focusing on slow, deep breaths.

2. **4-7-8 Breathing Technique**:

   - Sit or lie down comfortably.

   - Inhale through your nose for a count of 4.

   - Hold your breath for a count of 7.

   - Exhale completely through your mouth for a count of 8.

   - Repeat the cycle 4-8 times.

3. **Box Breathing**:

   - Inhale through your nose for a count of 4.

   - Hold your breath for a count of 4.

   - Exhale through your mouth for a count of 4.

   - Hold your breath for a count of 4.

   - Repeat the cycle for several minutes.

4. **Alternate Nostril Breathing (Nadi Shodhana)**:

   - Sit comfortably with your spine straight.

   - Close your right nostril with your right thumb.

- Inhale deeply through your left nostril.

   - Close your left nostril with your right ring finger, release your right nostril, and exhale through the right nostril.

   - Inhale through the right nostril, close it, and exhale through the left nostril.

- Continue alternating for 5-10 minutes.

Importance of Oxygen for Diabetes

1. **Cellular Metabolism**:

   - **Energy Production**: Oxygen is crucial for cellular respiration, the process by which cells produce energy. Efficient energy production helps in maintaining overall cellular health and function.

2. **Tissue Repair and Healing**:

   - **Improved Healing**: Adequate oxygen levels promote better healing and repair of tissues, which is particularly important for individuals with diabetes who may have delayed wound healing.

3. **Reduced Oxidative Stress**:

   - **Antioxidant Defense**: Proper oxygenation supports the body's antioxidant defense system, reducing oxidative stress and inflammation, which are linked to diabetes complications.

Potential Changes with Increased Oxygen:

- **Enhanced Glucose Metabolism**: Improved oxygenation can enhance cellular glucose uptake and metabolism, potentially leading to better blood sugar control.

- **Reduced Risk of Complications**: Adequate oxygen levels can help mitigate the risk of complications such as diabetic neuropathy and retinopathy by improving overall cellular health.

- **Improved Physical Performance**: Better oxygenation can lead to increased energy levels and improved physical performance, encouraging a more active lifestyle which is beneficial for diabetes management.

Conclusion:

Breathing exercises can be a valuable addition to diabetes management by reducing stress, improving oxygenation, and enhancing overall well-being. While breathing exercises alone are not a cure for diabetes, they can complement other treatments and lifestyle changes to help manage the condition more effectively. Individuals with diabetes should consult with their healthcare providers before starting any new exercise regimen, including breathing exercises.

Example Book Titles on Breathing Exercises for Diabetes:

1. **"Breathe Easy: Breathing Exercises for Better Diabetes Management"**

2. **"Oxygen and Diabetes: Harnessing Breathing Techniques for Health"**

3. **"The Diabetic's Guide to Breathing: Techniques for Improved Blood Sugar Control"**

4. **"Breath and Balance: Integrating Breathing Exercises into Diabetes Care"**

5. **"The Power of Breath: How Oxygen Therapy Can Help Manage Diabetes"**

These titles can provide comprehensive guidance on incorporating breathing exercises into diabetes management routines.

CHAPTER : 7

Nutrition and Diet

Importance of a Healthy Diet

In the world of diabetes management, one of the most crucial aspects to focus on is maintaining a healthy diet. A healthy diet plays a key role in managing blood sugar levels, reducing the risk of complications, and improving overall health. By understanding the importance of a healthy diet, individuals with diabetes can take control of their condition and improve their quality of life.

A healthy diet for individuals with diabetes should focus on balancing carbohydrates, proteins, and fats. By choosing whole, unprocessed foods such as fruits, vegetables, whole grains, lean proteins, and healthy fats, individuals can help keep their blood sugar levels stable and avoid spikes and crashes. Additionally, a healthy diet can help with weight management, which is important for controlling diabetes and reducing the risk of complications such as heart disease and stroke.

Incorporating a variety of nutrients into your diet is also crucial for overall health and well-being. Essential nutrients such as vitamins, minerals, and antioxidants play a key role in supporting the immune system, reducing inflammation, and promoting overall health. By choosing a wide range of colorful fruits and vegetables, individuals can ensure they are getting a diverse array of nutrients that will support their body's needs.

In addition to managing blood sugar levels and supporting overall health, a healthy diet can also help individuals with diabetes feel their best. Eating nutrient-dense foods can provide sustained energy levels, improve mental clarity, and support a healthy weight. By fueling the body with the right nutrients, individuals can experience improved focus, concentration, and mood, which can have a positive impact on their overall quality of life.

Overall, the importance of a healthy diet for individuals with diabetes cannot be overstated. By focusing on whole, unprocessed foods, balancing macronutrients, incorporating a variety of nutrients, and supporting overall health and well-being, individuals can take control of their condition and improve their quality of life. With the right approach to nutrition, individuals with diabetes can effectively manage their blood sugar levels, reduce the risk of complications, and live a healthy, fulfilling life.

Foods to Eat for Managing Diabetes

Managing diabetes through diet is crucial for maintaining optimal blood sugar levels and preventing complications. Choosing the right foods can help regulate blood sugar and improve overall health. Here are some key foods to incorporate into your diet to effectively manage diabetes.

1. Non-starchy vegetables: Non-starchy vegetables are low in calories and carbohydrates, making them an excellent choice for diabetes management. Vegetables such as leafy greens, broccoli, cauliflower, and bell peppers are rich in essential nutrients, fiber, and antioxidants. These vegetables can help control blood sugar levels and promote weight loss, which is essential for managing diabetes.

2. Whole grains: Whole grains are a great source of complex carbohydrates, which are digested more slowly than refined carbohydrates. This results in a gradual rise in blood sugar levels, making whole grains a better choice for diabetes management. Foods like brown rice, quinoa, oats, and whole wheat bread are high in fiber and nutrients, making them a healthy addition to your diet.

3. Lean protein: Protein is essential for stabilizing blood sugar levels and promoting satiety. Lean protein sources such as chicken, fish, tofu, and legumes can help regulate blood sugar and prevent spikes. Including protein in every meal can also help maintain muscle mass and support overall health in diabetes patients.

4. Healthy fats: Healthy fats are important for heart health and can help improve insulin sensitivity in diabetes patients. Foods like avocados, nuts, seeds, and olive oil are rich in monounsaturated fats, which can help reduce inflammation and improve blood sugar control. Including these fats in moderation can support a balanced diet and promote better diabetes management.

5. Fruits: While fruits contain natural sugars, they are also rich in fiber, vitamins, and antioxidants that can benefit diabetes patients. Choosing low-glycemic fruits like berries, apples, and citrus fruits can help regulate blood sugar levels and provide essential nutrients. Moderation is key when consuming fruits, as portion control can help prevent blood sugar spikes in diabetes patients.

Incorporating these key foods into your diet can help effectively manage diabetes and improve overall health. Remember to work with a healthcare provider or registered dietitian to create a personalized meal plan that meets your individual needs and goals. By making informed choices about the foods you eat, you can take control of your diabetes and lead a healthier, more fulfilling life.

Foods to Avoid for Managing Diabetes

When managing diabetes, it is crucial to pay close attention to the types of foods you consume. Some foods can cause blood sugar levels to spike, which can be harmful for individuals with diabetes. In this subchapter, we will discuss some of the foods that should be avoided in order to effectively manage diabetes and maintain optimal health.

One of the top foods to avoid for managing diabetes is sugary beverages, such as soda, fruit juice, and energy drinks. These drinks are loaded with sugar and can cause a rapid increase in blood sugar levels. It is best to opt for water, unsweetened tea, or other low-sugar options to stay hydrated and keep blood sugar levels stable.

Another food to avoid for managing diabetes is white bread and other refined grains. These foods are quickly broken down into sugar in the body, leading to spikes in blood sugar levels. Instead, choose whole grains like brown rice, quinoa, and whole wheat bread, which are higher in fiber and can help regulate blood sugar levels.

Processed foods, such as fast food, fried foods, and packaged snacks, should also be limited when managing diabetes. These foods are often high in unhealthy fats, added sugars, and salt, which can all negatively impact blood sugar levels and overall health. Opt for whole, unprocessed foods like fruits, vegetables, lean proteins, and nuts to support optimal diabetes management.

High-sugar desserts like cakes, cookies, and ice cream should be enjoyed in moderation or avoided altogether when managing diabetes. These treats can cause blood sugar levels to skyrocket and can lead to weight gain and other health complications. Instead, try satisfying your sweet tooth with fresh fruit, yogurt, or a small piece of dark chocolate to keep blood sugar levels in check.

Lastly, it is important to limit your intake of alcohol when managing diabetes. Alcohol can cause blood sugar levels to fluctuate, especially if consumed on an empty stomach or in excess. If you choose to drink, do so in moderation and be mindful of how it affects your blood sugar levels. Overall, making mindful food choices and avoiding these common culprits can help you effectively manage your diabetes and support your overall health and well-being.

CHAPTER : 8

Exercise and Physical Activity

Benefits of Exercise for Diabetes Management

Regular exercise is a crucial component of managing diabetes effectively. Not only does exercise help to control blood sugar levels, but it also plays a key role in improving overall health and reducing the risk of complications associated with diabetes. By incorporating regular physical activity into your daily routine, you can better manage your diabetes and improve your quality of life.

One of the primary benefits of exercise for diabetes management is its ability to lower blood sugar levels. When you engage in physical activity, your muscles use glucose for energy, which helps to reduce the amount of sugar in your bloodstream. This can help to prevent spikes in blood sugar levels and improve overall insulin sensitivity, making it easier for your body to regulate blood sugar effectively.

In addition to lowering blood sugar levels, regular exercise can also help to improve cardiovascular health, which is particularly important for individuals with diabetes. By engaging in activities that strengthen the heart and improve circulation, you can reduce your risk of heart disease and other complications associated with diabetes. Exercise can also help to lower blood pressure and cholesterol levels, further reducing the risk of cardiovascular problems.

Another key benefit of exercise for diabetes management is its ability to promote weight loss and improve body composition. Maintaining a healthy weight is essential for managing diabetes effectively, as excess weight can make it more difficult for your body to regulate blood sugar levels. By incorporating regular exercise into your routine, you can burn calories, build muscle, and improve your overall body composition, making it easier to manage your diabetes and maintain a healthy weight.

Overall, the benefits of exercise for diabetes management are numerous and significant. By making physical activity a regular part of your routine, you can lower blood sugar levels, improve cardiovascular health, promote weight loss, and reduce the risk of complications associated with diabetes. Whether you prefer walking, cycling, swimming, or another form of exercise, finding activities that you enjoy and incorporating them into your daily life can have a profound impact on your diabetes management and overall health.

Types of Physical Activity for Diabetes Patients

For individuals with diabetes, incorporating regular physical activity into their daily routine is crucial for effectively managing their condition. There are various types of physical activities that can benefit diabetes patients, helping to improve blood sugar levels, reduce the risk of complications, and enhance overall health and well-being. In this subchapter, we will explore different types of physical activity that are particularly beneficial for diabetes patients.

One type of physical activity that is highly recommended for diabetes patients is aerobic exercise. Aerobic activities, such as walking, running, cycling, swimming, and dancing, help to improve cardiovascular health, increase insulin sensitivity, and lower blood sugar levels. Aim for at least 150 minutes of moderate-intensity aerobic exercise per week, spread out over several days, to experience the benefits of aerobic exercise for diabetes management.

Another type of physical activity that can be beneficial for diabetes patients is strength training. Strength training exercises, such as weightlifting, bodyweight exercises, and resistance band workouts, help to build muscle mass, improve insulin sensitivity, and enhance overall physical strength and endurance. Incorporating strength training exercises into your routine at least two to three times per week can have a positive impact on your diabetes management.

Flexibility exercises, such as yoga and stretching, are also important for diabetes patients. These types of exercises help to improve flexibility, range of motion, and joint health, which can be especially beneficial for individuals with diabetes who may experience complications such as neuropathy or reduced circulation. Including flexibility exercises in your weekly routine can help to improve overall physical function and reduce the risk of injury.

Lastly, balance exercises are important for diabetes patients, particularly older adults who may be at risk of falls and injuries. Balance exercises, such as tai chi, Pilates, and balance drills, help to improve stability, coordination, and proprioception, reducing the risk of falls and enhancing overall physical confidence. Incorporating balance exercises into your routine can help to improve your quality of life and reduce the risk of injuries associated with diabetes-related complications.

In conclusion, there are various types of physical activity that can benefit diabetes patients, including aerobic exercise, strength training, flexibility exercises, and balance exercises. By incorporating a combination of these different types of physical activity into your routine, you can effectively manage your diabetes, improve your overall health and well-being, and reduce the risk of complications associated with the condition. Consult with your healthcare provider or a certified exercise specialist to create a personalized physical activity plan that meets your individual needs and goals.

Creating an Exercise Plan

Creating an exercise plan is a crucial component of effectively managing diabetes. Regular physical activity can help lower blood sugar levels, improve insulin sensitivity, and reduce the risk of complications associated with diabetes. When creating an exercise plan, it is important to consider your current fitness level, any health conditions you may have, and your overall goals for managing diabetes.

Start by consulting with your healthcare provider before beginning any new exercise regimen. They can help you determine a safe and effective exercise plan based on your individual needs and health status. Your healthcare provider may also recommend working with a certified diabetes educator or a personal trainer who has experience working with individuals with diabetes.

When creating your exercise plan, consider incorporating a mix of aerobic exercise, strength training, and flexibility exercises. Aerobic exercise, such as walking, swimming, or cycling, can help improve cardiovascular health and lower blood sugar levels. Strength training exercises, such as weight lifting or resistance band exercises, can help increase muscle mass and improve insulin sensitivity. Flexibility exercises, such as yoga or stretching, can help improve range of motion and prevent injury.

Set realistic and achievable goals for your exercise plan. Start with small, manageable goals and gradually increase the intensity and duration of your workouts as you become more comfortable and confident. Keep track of your progress and make adjustments to your exercise plan as needed. Remember that consistency is key when it comes to managing diabetes through exercise.

Incorporating regular physical activity into your daily routine can have a positive impact on your overall health and well-being. By creating an exercise plan that is tailored to your individual needs and goals, you can effectively manage diabetes and improve your quality of life. Remember to listen to your body, stay hydrated, and monitor your blood sugar levels before and after exercise to ensure your safety and success in managing diabetes.

CHAPTER : 9

Managing Stress and Mental Health

Impact of Stress on Blood Sugar Levels

Stress is a common factor that can have a significant impact on blood sugar levels for individuals living with diabetes. When the body experiences stress, it releases hormones such as cortisol and adrenaline, which can cause blood sugar levels to rise. This can be particularly problematic for individuals with diabetes, as it can make it more difficult to manage their condition effectively.

Research has shown that stress can lead to insulin resistance, where the body's cells are less responsive to insulin, the hormone responsible for regulating blood sugar levels. This means that even if a person with diabetes is taking insulin or other medications to manage their blood sugar, stress can still cause fluctuations in their levels. It is important for individuals with diabetes to be aware of the impact that stress can have on their blood sugar levels and to take steps to manage stress effectively.

One of the ways to combat the effects of stress on blood sugar levels is through stress management techniques such as meditation, deep breathing exercises, and regular physical activity. These activities can help to reduce the body's stress response and improve insulin sensitivity, making it easier to control blood sugar levels. Additionally, maintaining a healthy lifestyle with a balanced diet and regular exercise can also help to mitigate the effects of stress on blood sugar levels.

It is important for individuals with diabetes to be proactive in managing their stress levels in order to maintain stable blood sugar levels. This may involve seeking support from healthcare professionals, joining support groups, or practicing relaxation techniques on a regular basis. By taking steps to manage stress effectively, individuals with diabetes can improve their overall health and well-being, and better control their blood sugar levels.

In conclusion, stress can have a significant impact on blood sugar levels for individuals with diabetes, making it more challenging to manage their condition effectively. By understanding the relationship between stress and blood sugar levels, and implementing stress management techniques into their daily routine, individuals with diabetes can improve their overall health and well-being. It is essential for individuals with diabetes to prioritize their mental and emotional health in order to effectively manage their condition and minimize the impact of stress on their blood sugar levels.

Coping Strategies for Managing Stress

Living with diabetes can be a challenging experience, as the daily management of the condition can often lead to feelings of stress and overwhelm. However, there are several coping strategies that can help individuals effectively manage their stress levels and improve their overall well-being. By implementing these strategies, individuals can better navigate the complexities of living with diabetes and experience a higher quality of life.

One effective coping strategy for managing stress is to practice mindfulness and relaxation techniques. Mindfulness involves being fully present in the moment and can help individuals cultivate a sense of calm and inner peace. Techniques such as deep breathing exercises, meditation, and gentle yoga can all help reduce stress levels and promote relaxation. By incorporating these practices into their daily routine, individuals can better cope with the challenges of living with diabetes.

Another helpful coping strategy for managing stress is to engage in regular physical activity. Exercise has been shown to have numerous benefits for individuals with diabetes, including improved blood sugar control and reduced risk of complications. Additionally, physical activity can help reduce stress levels by releasing endorphins, which are chemicals in the brain that act as natural mood lifters. By incorporating regular exercise into their routine, individuals can better manage their stress levels and improve their overall well-being.

In addition to mindfulness and physical activity, it is important for individuals with diabetes to prioritize self-care and make time for activities that bring them joy. Engaging in hobbies, spending time with loved ones, and practicing self-care rituals can all help individuals reduce stress and improve their mental health. By making time for activities that bring them happiness and fulfillment, individuals can better cope with the challenges of living with diabetes and improve their overall quality of life.

Lastly, it is important for individuals with diabetes to seek support from their healthcare team, as well as from friends and family members. Talking to a healthcare provider about stress management techniques, attending support groups, and confiding in loved ones can all help individuals better cope with the challenges of living with diabetes. By seeking support from others, individuals can feel less alone in their journey and better navigate the complexities of managing their condition. By implementing these coping strategies, individuals with diabetes can effectively manage their stress levels and improve their overall well-being.

Importance of Mental Health Support

Mental health support is a crucial component of effectively managing diabetes. Living with a chronic illness like diabetes can take a toll on your mental well-being, leading to increased stress, anxiety, and even depression. By seeking out mental health support, you can learn coping strategies to better manage the emotional challenges that come with managing your diabetes. This can ultimately lead to improved overall health outcomes and a better quality of life.

One of the key benefits of mental health support for diabetes patients is the ability to reduce stress levels. Stress can have a significant impact on blood sugar levels, making it more difficult to control your diabetes. By learning stress management techniques through therapy or counseling, you can better regulate your blood sugar levels and improve your overall health. Additionally, reducing stress can lead to better sleep, improved mood, and increased energy levels.

Another important aspect of mental health support for diabetes patients is the ability to address any underlying issues that may be contributing to poor diabetes management. For example, individuals with a history of trauma or abuse may struggle with self-care and adherence to their diabetes treatment plan. By working with a mental health professional, you can address these underlying issues and develop strategies to overcome barriers to effective diabetes management.

In addition to reducing stress and addressing underlying issues, mental health support can also provide diabetes patients with a much-needed support system. Managing a chronic illness like diabetes can be isolating, and having a therapist or counselor to talk to can provide a sense of connection and understanding. This support can help you feel less alone in your journey with diabetes and provide encouragement and motivation to stay on track with your treatment plan.

Overall, mental health support is an essential component of effectively managing diabetes. By seeking out therapy, counseling, or other forms of mental health support, you can reduce stress, address underlying issues, and build a strong support system to help you navigate the challenges of living with diabetes. Remember, taking care of your mental health is just as important as taking care of your physical health when it comes to managing diabetes.

CHAPTER : 10

Complications and Prevention

Common Complications of Diabetes

Diabetes is a chronic condition that affects millions of people worldwide. While it can be effectively managed with proper treatment and lifestyle changes, there are also common complications that can arise if the condition is not well-controlled. In this sub-chapter, we will discuss some of the most common complications of diabetes and how they can be prevented or managed.

One of the most common complications of diabetes is diabetic neuropathy, which is nerve damage that can occur as a result of high blood sugar levels over time. This condition can cause pain, tingling, and numbness in the hands and feet, as well as digestive issues and sexual dysfunction. To prevent diabetic neuropathy, it is important to keep blood sugar levels under control through medication, diet, and exercise.

Another common complication of diabetes is diabetic retinopathy, which is damage to the blood vessels in the retina that can lead to vision loss. Regular eye exams and blood sugar monitoring are essential for preventing and managing diabetic retinopathy. In some cases, laser surgery may be necessary to treat the condition and preserve vision.

Diabetes can also increase the risk of heart disease and stroke, as high blood sugar levels can damage the blood vessels and lead to atherosclerosis. To reduce this risk, it is important for diabetes patients to maintain a healthy lifestyle, including eating a balanced diet, exercising regularly, and not smoking. Medications to control blood pressure and cholesterol levels may also be necessary.

Kidney disease is another common complication of diabetes, as high blood sugar levels can damage the kidneys over time. To prevent kidney disease, it is important to control blood sugar levels and blood pressure, as well as to avoid excessive alcohol consumption and maintain a healthy weight. In some cases, medications may be necessary to protect the kidneys from further damage.

Finally, diabetes can also increase the risk of infections and slow wound healing, as high blood sugar levels can weaken the immune system. To prevent infections and promote healing, it is important for diabetes patients to practice good hygiene, monitor blood sugar levels closely, and seek medical attention for any wounds that are slow to heal. By being proactive in managing their diabetes and addressing any complications that arise, patients can maintain their overall health and well-being.

Preventing Complications

Preventing complications is a crucial aspect of managing diabetes effectively. By taking proactive steps to monitor your blood sugar levels, follow a healthy diet, and maintain a regular exercise routine, you can significantly reduce your risk of developing complications associated with diabetes. One of the most important things you can do to prevent complications is to consistently monitor your blood sugar levels. By regularly checking your blood sugar levels throughout the day, you can ensure that they remain within a healthy range and take action if they start to spike or drop.

Additionally, following a healthy diet is essential for preventing complications associated with diabetes. A diet rich in fruits, vegetables, whole grains, and lean proteins can help you maintain stable blood sugar levels and reduce your risk of developing complications such as heart disease, nerve damage, and vision problems. It's also important to limit your intake of sugary and processed foods, as these can cause your blood sugar levels to spike and lead to complications over time.

In addition to monitoring your blood sugar levels and following a healthy diet, regular exercise is another key component of preventing complications associated with diabetes. Exercise not only helps you maintain a healthy weight, but it also improves your body's ability to regulate blood sugar levels and reduces your risk of developing complications such as heart disease and nerve damage. Aim to incorporate at least 30 minutes of moderate-intensity exercise into your daily routine, such as walking, cycling, or swimming, to reap the benefits of physical activity.

Furthermore, it's important to work closely with your healthcare team to develop a comprehensive treatment plan that addresses your individual needs and goals. By regularly seeing your doctor, diabetes educator, and other healthcare providers, you can stay informed about your condition and make any necessary adjustments to your treatment plan to prevent complications. Your healthcare team can also provide guidance on managing stress, quitting smoking, and other lifestyle factors that can impact your diabetes management and overall health.

In conclusion, preventing complications associated with diabetes requires a proactive approach to managing your condition. By monitoring your blood sugar levels, following a healthy diet, maintaining a regular exercise routine, and working closely with your healthcare team, you can reduce your risk of developing complications and improve your overall quality of life. Remember that managing diabetes is a lifelong journey, but with the right strategies and support, you can effectively prevent complications and master your diabetes.

Regular Check-ups and Monitoring

Regular check-ups and monitoring are essential components of effectively managing diabetes. As a diabetes patient, it is crucial to stay on top of your health by scheduling routine appointments with your healthcare provider. These check-ups allow for the monitoring of your blood sugar levels, as well as the evaluation of your overall health and the effectiveness of your current treatment plan.

During these appointments, your healthcare provider will conduct various tests to assess your diabetes management. This may include measuring your blood sugar levels, checking your blood pressure, and performing a physical examination. By regularly monitoring these key indicators, your healthcare provider can make adjustments to your treatment plan as needed to ensure that your diabetes is well-managed.

In addition to regular check-ups with your healthcare provider, self-monitoring is also an important aspect of managing diabetes. This may involve checking your blood sugar levels at home using a glucometer, keeping track of your diet and exercise habits, and monitoring for any symptoms of complications related to diabetes. By staying vigilant and proactive in monitoring your health, you can better understand how your body responds to different factors and make informed decisions about your diabetes management.

It is important to communicate openly and honestly with your healthcare provider during regular check-ups. Be sure to discuss any concerns or questions you may have about your diabetes management, as well as any changes in your symptoms or overall health. Your healthcare provider is there to support you and work with you to develop a personalized treatment plan that meets your specific needs and goals.

By prioritizing regular check-ups and monitoring as part of your diabetes management plan, you can take control of your health and work towards mastering diabetes. Remember that consistency is key, and by staying proactive and engaged in your healthcare, you can effectively manage your diabetes and live a healthy, fulfilling life.

CHAPTER : 11

Resources and Support

Support Groups for Diabetes Patients

Support groups for diabetes patients can be incredibly beneficial for those navigating the challenges of managing their condition. These groups provide a safe and understanding space where individuals can share their experiences, gain valuable insights, and receive emotional support from others who are facing similar struggles. By connecting with others who are also dealing with diabetes, patients can feel less alone in their journey and build a sense of community that can be empowering and uplifting.

One of the key benefits of joining a support group for diabetes patients is the opportunity to learn from the experiences of others. Members can share tips, strategies, and resources that have been helpful in managing their diabetes effectively. This exchange of information can be invaluable for individuals looking to improve their own self-care practices and make informed decisions about their treatment plan. By tapping into the collective wisdom of the group, patients can gain new perspectives and insights that can enhance their overall quality of life.

In addition to providing practical advice and support, diabetes support groups also offer a unique opportunity for emotional connection and validation. Living with a chronic condition like diabetes can be emotionally taxing, and it's common for patients to experience feelings of isolation, frustration, and anxiety. In a support group setting, individuals can openly discuss their feelings and concerns with others who truly understand what they are going through. This sense of camaraderie can help reduce feelings of loneliness and provide a sense of belonging that can be incredibly comforting.

Another important aspect of support groups for diabetes patients is the sense of accountability that comes from being part of a community. By regularly attending meetings and engaging with other members, patients can stay motivated and committed to their self-care routine. Knowing that others are counting on them can be a powerful motivator for sticking to healthy habits, such as monitoring blood sugar levels, following a balanced diet, and staying active. This accountability can help individuals stay on track with their treatment plan and achieve better health outcomes in the long run.

Overall, joining a support group for diabetes patients can be a valuable resource for individuals looking to effectively manage their condition and improve their quality of life. By connecting with others who share similar experiences, patients can gain practical advice, emotional support, and a sense of community that can be truly transformative. Whether you are newly diagnosed with diabetes or have been living with the condition for years, consider exploring the benefits of joining a support group to enhance your journey towards mastering diabetes.

Online Resources for Managing Diabetes

Managing diabetes can be a complex and challenging task, but thanks to the wealth of online resources available today, patients have access to a wealth of information and support to help them navigate their condition. Whether you are newly diagnosed or have been living with diabetes for years, the internet offers a plethora of tools and resources to help you manage your diabetes effectively.

One of the most valuable online resources for diabetes management is the plethora of educational websites dedicated to providing up-to-date information on the latest research, treatment options, and lifestyle strategies for managing diabetes. Websites such as the American Diabetes Association, Diabetes UK, and Beyond Type 1 offer a wealth of resources, from articles and guides to forums and support groups where patients can connect with others who are facing similar challenges.

In addition to educational websites, there are also numerous apps and online tools available to help patients track their blood sugar levels, monitor their diet and exercise habits, and stay on top of their medication regimen. Apps like MySugr, Glucose Buddy, and MyFitnessPal can be invaluable tools for managing diabetes on the go, allowing patients to easily track their progress and stay motivated to make healthy choices.

For patients who prefer a more personalized approach to diabetes management, online coaching programs and telemedicine services can provide individualized support and guidance from diabetes experts. These programs often include one-on-one coaching sessions, personalized meal plans, and ongoing support to help patients achieve their health goals and improve their diabetes management.

Overall, the internet offers a treasure trove of resources for diabetes patients looking to take control of their health and manage their condition effectively. By taking advantage of these online tools and resources, patients can empower themselves with the knowledge and support they need to live well with diabetes and minimize the risk of complications. Whether you are looking for information, support, or personalized guidance, the online world is a valuable resource for mastering diabetes and achieving optimal health.

Finding a Healthcare Team

Finding a healthcare team to support you in managing your diabetes is an essential step in effectively navigating your diagnosis. A strong healthcare team can provide you with the guidance, resources, and support needed to successfully manage your diabetes and improve your overall health. When seeking out a healthcare team, it's important to consider the expertise and experience of each member to ensure that you receive the best possible care.

One key member of your healthcare team should be a primary care physician or endocrinologist who specializes in diabetes management. These healthcare providers can help you monitor your blood sugar levels, adjust your medication as needed, and provide guidance on lifestyle changes that can improve your diabetes management. Additionally, a registered dietitian can help you create a meal plan that supports your diabetes management goals and ensures that you are getting the nutrients you need to stay healthy.

In addition to medical professionals, it's also important to include other specialists on your healthcare team who can help you manage the various aspects of diabetes. This may include a podiatrist to monitor your foot health, an ophthalmologist to check your eye health, and a mental health professional to support your emotional well-being. By assembling a comprehensive healthcare team, you can address all aspects of diabetes management and ensure that you receive the best possible care.

When selecting healthcare providers for your team, it's important to consider their communication style and how well they work with you as a patient. Building a strong relationship with your healthcare team is crucial for effective diabetes management, as it allows for open communication, mutual respect, and collaboration in developing a personalized treatment plan. Be sure to ask questions, voice your concerns, and actively participate in your healthcare decisions to ensure that you are receiving the best possible care.

Overall, finding a healthcare team that supports and guides you in managing your diabetes is essential for your overall health and well-being. By assembling a team of medical professionals who specialize in diabetes management, as well as other specialists who can address the various aspects of diabetes, you can take control of your diagnosis and work towards improved health outcomes. Remember to communicate openly with your healthcare team, actively participate in your care, and seek out support when needed to effectively manage your diabetes and live your best life.

Dear Readers,

Thank you for choosing to read **Ultimate Guide to Mastering Diabetes: Proven Strategies and Therapy for Effective Diagnosis and Management**. I hope this book has provided you with valuable insights and practical strategies to effectively manage and master diabetes.

Your feedback is incredibly important to me, and I would love to hear about your experience with the book. Please take a moment to leave a review on Amazon Kindle. Your honest thoughts and opinions will not only help me improve but also assist other readers in discovering how this book might help them in their journey to better health.

When writing your review, you might consider answering the following questions:

- How has this book impacted your understanding of diabetes management?

- Were the strategies and tips provided helpful and easy to implement?

- Did any particular section or chapter resonate with you or stand out?

- Would you recommend this book to others dealing with diabetes?

Thank you again for your support. Your review means a lot and contributes to the success of this book. I look forward to reading your thoughts!

Warm regards,

Bhupen Thapa

How to Leave a Review on Amazon Kindle:

1. Go to the product page for **Ultimate Guide to Mastering Diabetes: Proven Strategies and Therapy for Effective Diagnosis and Management** on Amazon.

2. Scroll down to the "Customer Reviews" section.

3. Click on the "Write a customer review" button.

4. Rate the book from 1 to 5 stars and write your review in the provided text box.

5. Click "Submit" to post your review.

Thank you for taking the time to share your thoughts!